How to Help
Friends & Family
Through
Infertility

How to Help
Friends & Family
Through
Infertility

How You Can Offer Support, What To Say, and Understanding Infertility

ALEXANDRA KORNSWIET

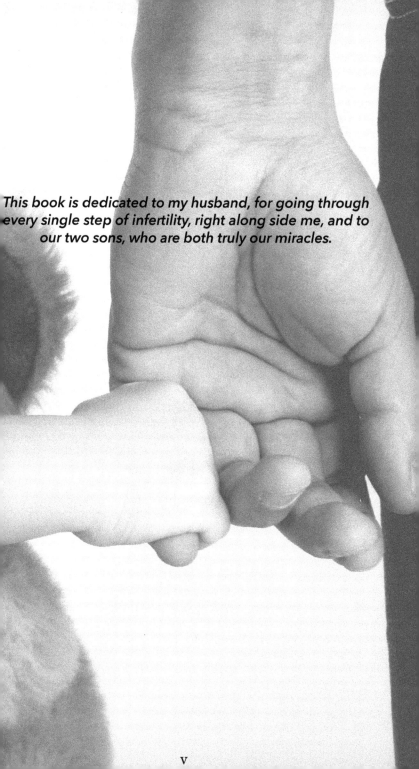

This book is dedicated to my husband, for going through every single step of infertility, right along side me, and to our two sons, who are both truly our miracles.

Table of Contents

Introduction

Introduction

Who Am I?

I'm Alex. My husband and I have been dealing with infertility since 2015. It is something that has become a huge part of our lives and is something I am incredibly passionate about helping others through. We are high school sweethearts who started dating in 2005, at age sixteen and seventeen respectively, and have been together ever since. We got married in 2012 and decided we wanted to start a family in 2015. Prior to trying to start our family, we had lived in many different places together, including a summer in Hong Kong, and we were lucky enough to travel a good amount together as well. We felt we had experienced so much as a couple, and we could not wait to start our family together. Like many others, we had no idea where our path would lead.

Although this book is about infertility, that is not the only part of me. I am also a mother, a wife, a daughter, a friend, a sister, a granddaughter, a baker, and more. I worked in bakeries and hotels for years and moved to different management positions after that. I always thought I wanted to own my own bakery, and it is still a long-term dream for my husband and me, but for now, I have found a passion in advocacy, community, and education for infertility.

Why Did I Write This Book?

I never expected to be part of the world of infertility and the infertility community, but now that I am, I am extremely passionate about not only helping people get the support they need but also helping people offer support to those who need it. I wrote this book for those who want to offer support, but do not know how. It can feel isolating to be the support person sometimes because you never feel like you are saying the right thing. While I know it is impossible to completely understand what someone is going through without experiencing it yourself, I do think it is possible to learn how to support someone in a way that will be beneficial and helpful to both you and them. This book is a series of suggestions, reminders, and education to help you feel better prepared to support your friends and family experiencing infertility.

Why Should You Read It?

You should read it if you want to support a friend or family member through infertility. Even if you think you know how, I truly believe you will gain something from this book as a whole. Remember, just by picking up this book, you are showing that you want to help, and you want to offer support. You are already well intentioned, and even if you have done or not done something outlined below, that does not mean you are not a good person. You are a wonderful person, but it is also natural not to know how to support someone when you have not personally experienced what they have. I offer suggestions of how to phrase your language, how to offer support, and when to offer support. I also give reminders for what it feels like to be the person experiencing infertility, and why we often react (or do not react) the way we do. The final section of the book is more technical, and focuses on the logistics of what infertility is, what treatment options are, and more. This is aimed to give you more background so you can better understand the details of what your friend or family member may be experiencing daily. If you want a perspective of someone who has and is experiencing infertility, miscarriage, and more, you have come to the right place! I promise that getting the perspective from someone who has experienced it can only be helpful.

i've built more
relationships
with people
by being open
about my struggles
than I ever could
have pretending
like I had it all
together.

Be Patient

Be Patient

I wanted to start with this chapter because infertility is a long road, and there is a lot to process. So please be patient with those experiencing infertility and try to remember they are navigating a very challenging path.

There Are Many Things to Mourn

Infertility includes a giant lack of control over something that should be basic and simple, having children. And with that lack of control comes uncertainty, fear of the unknown, and more. When your friend or family member found out they were suffering from infertility, they had to mourn a natural path to children that they assumed would happen for them, as most do. And they have to continue to mourn different outcomes or possibilities along the way.

For those trying naturally, they may be mourning a negative pregnancy test each month or a period that comes when they are hoping it finally will not. It can be realizing that they will not get the surprise they were hoping for, while they carefully track every moment of each month, consumed by waiting for good news to finally come. For those who cannot try naturally, experiencing infertility can mean they will never be able to just take a test and have it be positive. It can be not having the opportunity to surprise friends and family with the news, since many usually know what is going on. And for those doing fertility treatments, the mourning can be for cancelled cycles, failed transfers, miscarriages, and more.

A loss is a loss. And every loss is painful and needs to be grieved. Many people going through infertility will experience multiple types of loss throughout their journeys, and will need to continue to mourn different aspects throughout. Be patient as they do this, and continue to be there for them. And please, do not compare these losses to simply not getting pregnant after trying for a single month. All of these losses are devastating. This experience involves time, energy, money, and emotional and physical aspects—and they all cumulate in very challenging moments.

It Is About Them, Not You

At the end of the day, remember that a person's infertility, and their path and desire to have a child or children, is about them, not you. It can be confusing because sometimes they might be more open to sharing, while at other times feel more reserved and shut off. Every day is different, and they probably do not even know how they will be feeling about it from one day to the next. Respect if they want to share, but also respect if they do not. And if they have shared something before, that is not an open invitation to questions and comments forever. Respect the fact that they may want space and may not want to talk at all sometimes. And if they do want to talk about it, it is great to really listen closely to what they are going through. They may not always want to give details, but you can still hear what is going on with them when they do talk about it—and you can do your own research if you are curious to know more. To help with that, I have included an entire chapter on researching infertility, so that may be a starting point to learn more about this process.

Since it can be confusing to know when or how to help a friend or family member experiencing infertility, one of the best things to do so is to ask them what they need, but respect if they just need space. Every person is different with how they process things, and people can change their minds, so just letting a person know you are there can mean so much. A simple check-in once in a while, a reminder that you are there if the person needs you, can mean the world and be all that they really need sometimes.

Forgive Them

I know it sounds strange to ask you to forgive the person in pain—but you may need to do this. It can be easy for someone suffering to take things out on you, to blame you for a misunderstanding, or to lash out when it is not your fault at all. Forgive your friend or family member for saying the wrong thing or acting the wrong way toward you. They are in a place of pain and uncertainty, and they may not know what they need or how to express it. They may be taking what you say personally even if you do not mean it. Please be patient, forgiving, and understanding, and know that they are just healing and trying to move through things in their own way.

This forgiveness may also extend to events or experiences they have missed with you or loved ones. Sometimes they may not be able to attend an event or show up for something. You should still invite them, to give them the option of coming or not, as they also would not want to feel excluded, but understand that sometimes they have to put their own well-being and mental health in front of supporting others. For example, if there is a baby shower that you expected them to go to, and they did not come, please understand that it may have been far too painful for them to attend. They wish it was not, but they had to protect themselves and take care of their own well-being first.

Healing Takes Time

When your friend or family member is healing from loss or mourning a change or disappointment, please remember that this can take time. No one's timeline is the same, and healing is not linear. Please do not expect them to be "over" something just because you have moved on and realize that these past pains and constant uncertainties are on their mind a lot more than yours. They would love to be able to just move forward and stop hurting, but this takes time, and they need the patience and understanding to do so in their own way.

Overall, it is important to respect the space of the person experiencing infertility and understand that it is not your fault— or theirs. They will heal in their own way, on their own time, and sometimes backtrack from that healing. Infertility can be a long, hard road, and just knowing you are there for them can be all someone needs.

Triggering Words

Triggering Words

When you are going through infertility, there are certain words or phrases that can be incredibly triggering, and they are not always obvious to people who are not going through it. These are sometimes the most common things that people say, usually out of love and support, but they can actually make people feel worse. This is not to say you are a bad person if you have used these words or phrases—you are human! I just want to point them out so that you can try to avoid saying them in the future and be more mindful about how the person you are trying to support processes your language.

"At Least"

The words "at least" can be a trigger. There is nothing "at least" about infertility. People often make the mistake of thinking that the best thing to do is to try to see the silver lining, but sometimes people just need to express their emotions and feelings and share what they have experienced without finding a bright spot. Yes, it is good to eventually start to hope again, but if someone is sharing their bad news with you, regardless of what it is, just listen. For example, if a younger person is suffering from infertility, do not say "at least you're young." Age does not equal fertility health, and it does not equal having children for sure, so this is not comforting. Instead, just say you are sorry for what they are going through, you know it must be so hard, and that you are there for them. Here are some other examples of hurtful phrases that start with these two words:

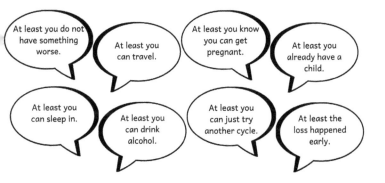

At least you do not have something worse.

At least you can travel.

At least you know you can get pregnant.

At least you already have a child.

At least you can sleep in.

At least you can drink alcohol.

At least you can just try another cycle.

At least the loss happened early.

People with infertility are still suffering, so it is not fair to compare it to something that potentially could be worse for them. This is already very hard for them. Also, someone with infertility would gladly give up travel, sleep, drinking, and more for a child —they are not grateful they can still do those things. For the phrases about getting pregnant, someone is trying to have a healthy child, not just get pregnant, and sometimes just because you can get pregnant does not mean you will ever actually have a child, so that is hurtful as well. Overall, all of these phrases dismiss everything your friend or family member has been through, and it makes them feel that everything they experienced is not enough. It makes them feel that they are not worthy of the pain they are feeling and do not deserve to mourn, when they absolutely do.

"Just"

"Just" is a trigger. It is a simple, small word—but it sure is a popular one to say to people struggling with infertility. Ultimately, it is usually the wrong thing to say. For example:

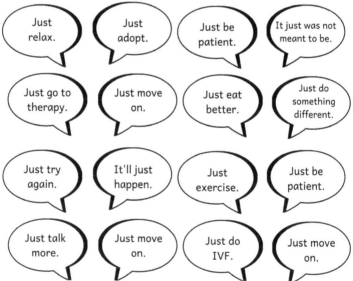

The list could go on and on, and instead of opinions, all your friend or loved one really needs is hugs, love, and support instead. Many times, we just need that.

"When" or "Why"

These are triggers on their own, because they lead to so many other questions.

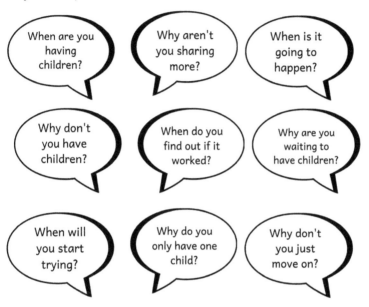

This lists just some of the examples, but overall, tread carefully with the personal questions you ask. These are so common for even strangers to say, and it can be extremely triggering and hurtful.

What To Say or Do Instead

These are just a few of the main categories of harmful phrases to avoid, but the key takeaway is that there are simpler, more meaningful, and kinder ways to respond to people going through infertility.

You can say: "I'm sorry", "That sucks", "I'm here for you", "I'm sorry for what you are going through". Or you can offer a hug or let them know you are there for support.

Those experiencing infertility do not want opinions. They do not want unsolicited advice. They do not want you to tell them how to do things or what they are doing right or wrong.

They just need support. They just need love. They just need hugs. They just need to know that it is okay if they are angry or upset or frustrated.

You do not need to fix it. They cannot fix it, so they do not expect you to. They just want to know they are not alone.

make
people
feel
loved
today

What Not
To Do

What Not To Do

Now that we have talked about words that can be triggering, here are some actions and suggestions that can be equally hurtful, along with suggestions of what to do instead.

1 Stop asking people when they are having children

This is an extremely triggering question, and way too common in our society. People assume it is okay to ask this to anyone and everyone, and the assumption is that everyone wants children, and that it will happen easily for anyone. Some people have children easily, some people have an incredibly difficult time, and some people do not want any children. If someone is already having a hard time dealing with the fact that they want a child or children so badly, they do not need the constant reminder that they do not have them. In addition to that, if someone does have a child, stop asking them how many they want or when they are going to have another child. That can be just as hurtful, as you do not know their situation and should not assume you do. So please, just think of something else to talk about. There is so much else to talk about.

2 Do not offer unsolicited advice

This can come in the form of suggesting new treatments, asking if someone has tried ___, telling them a new doctor to go to, telling them when to stop or when to keep going, and more. Instead just be there if they want to talk and understand when they do not. As I said before, you cannot fix infertility with your opinions, and no one is asking you to, so refrain from unsolicited advice. If someone is sharing something with you, it is not because they are seeking answers from you—it is simply that they are sharing. That is it. They do not need you to try to fix it. And besides, they have probably tried everything you can think of.

3 Do not tell a story about someone else you know just to relate to them

A lot of times people feel that the best way to support someone is by relating to them. And this often comes in the form of a story about someone they knew once, or heard of, who experienced something just like them. This is not the right way to offer support. It is downplaying what your friend or loved one is trying to talk about with you and taking the focus from them to you. Just listen. Just acknowledge that it is difficult for them. That is all they need.

4 Do not make something up or exaggerate an experience to relate

It is okay if you do not completely understand, and it is okay if you cannot really relate—the person experiencing infertility gets that, but please do not make up something or exaggerate just to try to relate to someone. For example, a "pregnancy scare" is not the same as a miscarriage. I am sorry if it happened, but you had a healthy baby, so please do not tell that story to say you understand the other person's loss. This also applies to pregnancy symptoms—even if you had a very hard pregnancy with a lot of morning sickness, it is still not the same as losing the pregnancy or not being able to have a child at all. Sometimes it can feel that talking about your experiences and relating are the best way to make someone else feel better but it really just points out that you have a child, when they still do not. So please, just refrain from doing this.

5 Do not ask whose "fault" it is or assume or know

This can be extremely hurtful, but it is a common question People want to know where the infertility stems from. But to us this does not matter. No matter who has the infertility issues, it is hard, and it is something both people in the relationship are going through.

6   Do not gossip about a friend's issues

When your friend or family member shares what they are going through and comes to you for support, please do not share it with anyone else. They are being vulnerable and expect your privacy and confidentiality. It is not your experience or your news to share; it is theirs. Unless they explicitly ask you to pass information along to others, assume it is confidential.

7   Do not just talk about babies, infertility, pregnancy, etc.

People going through infertility are already completely consumed by thoughts of babies, pregnancy, and infertility all day long, so one of the best ways to offer support is to talk about something completely unrelated! Do something together that has nothing to do with what they are experiencing—play a game, or just distract them overall. These distractions can feel very welcome and very appreciated!

8   Do not assume a friend is pregnant if you have not heard from them in a while

This can be a common thought, assumption, or question when you have not heard from someone in a while. They probably are not, and even if they are, it is not their job to share every aspect of their lives right away. They get to decide when to share, what to share, and how to share. And if they are pregnant, do not say that you "knew" it. They did not know it, so you definitely did not either. And this phrase can take away some of their joy from finally being able to share news with you. So please, think again before you say this.

Offer to Help
No Strings
Attached

Offer to Help, No Strings Attached

While your friend of family member may not always want to talk about what is going on with them, they will likely need your help and support in other ways. The problem is, they will feel like if they ask you for help, they may be obligated to share every detail of their experience with you, which can deter them from asking for your help. So please, offer to help, and explain that they do not need to give you any personal information in exchange. You simply want to help, with no strings attached.

1   Offer to attend an appointment

They may not say yes, and they may not be able to have you attend, but just offering can be extremely nice and show how much you care. Sometimes, just having someone to drive there with, while talking about something completely different, can help with anxiety. And if they would prefer to go alone, respect that answer too.

2   Offer to help with older kids

If your friend or family member already has children, they may need help with them while attending appointments or having treatments done. Offering to help them with their children, while expecting no explanations or information in exchange, is something they will be incredibly grateful for.

3   Accept boundaries

Sometimes your friend or family member will want to talk about it, but sometimes they will not. Really listen, and sometimes just listen, without advice, without ideas, without your own stories. Just listen and let them know you are there for them. And do not press for more information. If they want to share more, they will.

4   Simply check in

Just because your friend or family member is putting on a smile does not mean they are okay. They may be waiting for you to check in on them, just to ask how they are doing, or say you are thinking of them or there for them if they want to talk. Getting a text from a friend, without expecting a return text, can be very helpful. But with this said, please be mindful of when you ask them and how often you ask them. Usually a text is best, as being asked in person can put the spotlight on them, when they probably do not want to talk about it in front of others. There is also a chance they may not want to talk at all, so respect their response to you, even if they choose not to respond at all.

5   Ask how they want to be supported

Even though checking in can be extremely kind, not everyone wants to be asked if they are okay or contacted regularly. This counteracts the last point, but everyone is different. You can even text or email your friend or family member and ask how they prefer to be supported. This is very thoughtful and shows that you want to support them in a way that specifically helps them. But remember, listen to what they say and trust that they are telling you the truth. Please do not infer that they are leaving something out, or that they are holding back. If they say they do not want to talk about it, or that they do not want to be asked anymore, respect that! Trust me, they know what they want better than you do, so believe them when they tell you.

The most truly generous persons are those who give silently without hope or praise of reward.

CAROL RYRIE BRINK

How to Share Pregnancy News

How to Share
Pregnancy News

Pregnancy announcements can be extremely triggering. They can also cause feelings of shame. Often, those experiencing infertility so badly want only to be happy for friends and family who have good news, and they feel guilty when they think about themselves first. But how can they not? They often think about how they are still not pregnant or ask why it cannot happen to them too. In many cases, they can be genuinely happy for you but sad for themselves at the same time. Those feelings are not mutually exclusive; they live together. And while that is confusing, it is just part of dealing with infertility.

With that said, if you get pregnant and want to share the news with your infertile friend or family member, please do so with thoughtfulness. Here are ideas of how to share the news:

1   Give them space to react

For many people, the best way to hear the news is through a personal text or email. That way, they can react to it honestly, without feeling they are taking away from your happiness or good news. Do not expect them to respond right away and understand that their response may take time. I promise you it is not personal; they are just trying to process their feelings about what is happening (or not happening) to them too.

2   Understand that regardless of their reaction, they can be happy for you and sad for them

I said this before, but it is vital to remember. If they cannot support you in your happy times right away, do not take it personally. They could just be having a hard time keeping it together as it is. They can be happy for you and sad for themselves simultaneously.

3 Do not complain to them about your pregnancy

This should be obvious, but unfortunately it is not always. They wish they could feel sick, tired, or achy, or however you are feeling. They are putting their bodies through hell just in the hope that they will feel that way soon. Find someone else to complain to.

4 Tell them that you understand and support them

When you give your news, it is especially thoughtful if you call out the fact that you understand where they are coming from. Tell them that you respect whatever they need to process and heal. A wonderful example is on the next page. This is a real text I received from a very good friend, and I believe she handled it perfectly. No one wants to take away from your good news or your spotlight, but since your news is good, find other friends and family to share more excitement with.

5 Do not share other people's news

This should be obvious, but please do not share news about someone else's pregnancy, especially if your infertile friend does not even know them. It can be hard enough just to hear pregnancy announcements when it is a family member or friend, but it is even worse if the person experiencing infertility does not know the person. Some people share news to try to bring up situations of hope, which is understandable, but it is usually just another reminder that your friend or family member still is not the one with that is having a child. So please do not share this news with them if it is not necessary.

"Hey, wanted to share the news with you that I'm pregnant. We are planning to share the news with the rest of the group tonight but wanted to tell you first so that it didn't come out of nowhere. I know that hearing this kind of news from other people must be incredibly difficult. We love you guys so much - you are always on our hearts and minds. No need to respond to this if you don't want to. I don't want you to feel forced to express any emotions that don't feel right for you right now."

Infertility Affects Mental Health

Infertility Affects Mental Health

For many people, the physical aspects of infertility are the most obvious, followed by the financial aspects. While these are very important and vital to consider, mental health and the emotional aspects of infertility are often forgotten, or barely considered at all. Personally, and I believe many would agree with me, the emotional and mental aspects of infertility are the most difficult part. If only the desire for children was lifted from them, they would not be where they are, so the hope, the drive, the heartbreak, and more— that is what is so hard to cope with.

And the mental health aspect affects people before, during, and after infertility. No matter how someone's infertility journey ends (by choice or not), the mental aspects continue to affect a person far after the physical. One of the biggest mental aspects of infertility is infertility trauma. The trauma can be influenced by past experiences, experiences with infertility itself, and the aftermath of infertility.

Honestly, it took me a really long time to realize how much trauma impacts infertility. I felt it, but I did not have a name for it. Trauma. Traumatic. PTSD. Anxiety. Depression. Grief. Loss. It is part of infertility, and it is real. And people should not be ashamed of that, and they should not feel they have to hide it.

> "The mental health aspects continue to affect a person far after the physical..."

It affects them before, during, and after infertility, regardless of what their infertility resolution is—and they should be able to talk about it, talk through it, connect, and heal. And healing does not mean fixing, and it does not mean they will feel good forever or every single day —it means they are working through their feelings and their traumas, and they are accepting what has happened and what is real for them.

Prior to experiencing infertility, many of them have had other traumas or hard experiences in life, and infertility can bring these up again for them. There are so many uncertainties, so many unknowns, a giant lack of control, and so much more—of course it is a lot to go through! And even if they do have that child they have been yearning for, they can still face the traumas of infertility in unexpected moments.

So instead of pushing their feelings down, ignoring their past, or trying to push through things without acknowledging their experiences and traumas, I urge people to come together and support each other. It should be more acceptable to seek out help, to talk about how you are feeling, to express all ranges of emotions, and more. A person cannot truly heal or move on without acknowledging the mental health aspect of infertility.

One day you will tell your story of how you've overcome what you're going through now, and it will become part of someone else's survival guide.

Do Your Research

Do Your Research

Imagine this: You are twenty-six years old, newly married, and considering starting a family. You have always wanted children, and everyone in your family has been able to have as many as they want, whenever they want. It is assumed that when you are ready, it will happen. You start trying, and quickly you are overcome with the obsession to make it work. You are not just considering it now, you want children—and you want a child now. But something is not right. Something does not seem to be working. Months pass. You ask your doctor, and they tell you to relax. They tell you that it can just take time. You are young. It will happen. They guarantee it. But you know yourself—and something is not right. So, you advocate for yourself and find a doctor who will listen. And you were right—something is wrong. You have a physical issue that inhibits you from getting pregnant, unless you use in vitro fertilization (IVF). And this is a shock. You are blindsided but grateful you fought for yourself.

Of course, this did not happen you; this is what happened to me. And this is only my example—everyone's diagnoses and realization that they are experiencing infertility is different. Even my original doctor was wrong, so do not blame yourself if you do not know how to help people. That is where this book comes in.

Why Should I Do My Own Research?

Infertility is something that you are either completely engrossed in or completely oblivious to—there is usually not much of an in-between. As young children, we are taught to be afraid to get pregnant, but we are never taught that anyone has a difficult, or impossible, time having children. So when people first realize they are suffering from infertility, they feel blindsided. Treatments are introduced with no background or baseline. With that said, it makes sense that those supporting them know even less. If you have not been through it, why would you know anything about it? If it has not affected you, it is understandable that you do not know. But the person experiencing infertility may not want to be the one to explain

31

every step, so an incredible way you can offer support is to do your own research.

Remember, support and curiosity are not the same thing—most people going through infertility do not want to be there to educate you as well. This chapter is to help you understand more of the basics behind infertility and treatments so you can better understand, without asking the person going through it. They will also appreciate that you care enough to do your own research.

It can mean a lot to someone if you care about what they are specifically going through. They might not want to spend hours explaining everything they have been through, but they will appreciate it if you look into it on your own to try to understand them. Do you know if they are going through a treatment? Many treatments involve shots, and those shots can cause bruises or pain. Maybe something as simple as sending them an ice or heat pack can brighten their day. It means you considered something they need and were thoughtful enough to look into that yourself.

What Is Infertility?

First of all, infertility is a disease. It is a recognized, real disease, even though it is often not talked about as one. If you look up the technical definition, it is said to be "a disease of the reproductive system defined by the failure to achieve a clinical pregnancy after 12 months or more of regular unprotected sexual intercourse."[1] While I agree that it is absolutely a disease, I think this definition simplifies it. I was diagnosed after only trying for about six months, but many try for years before they get answers. I was only diagnosed earlier because I fought for myself, and found a doctor who would listen. Instead of sticking with this limited definition, I will explain more about what the possible diagnoses are, what possible treatment options are and more. The person you are trying to support may have mentioned something you see in this book, and now you will know more about it without having to ask them for details. They still might not want to share or might not want to discuss their particular issues in detail, but it is nice for you to do your own research. It is already a huge part of their life, and they may want to just be able to talk about other things sometimes.

What are the Possible Diagnoses for Infertility?

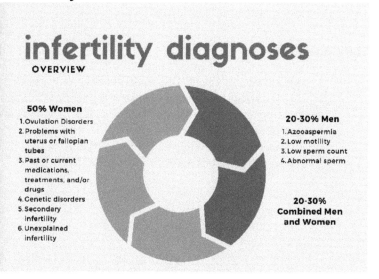

infertility diagnoses
OVERVIEW

50% Women
1. Ovulation Disorders
2. Problems with uterus or fallopian tubes
3. Past or current medications, treatments, and/or drugs
4. Genetic disorders
5. Secondary infertility
6. Unexplained infertility

20-30% Men
1. Azooaspermia
2. Low motility
3. Low sperm count
4. Abnormal sperm

20-30% Combined Men and Women

Infertility can affect anyone—it does not matter your gender, race, sexual orientation, spoken language, and so forth. It affects people everywhere. According to the Centers for Disease Control in the United States, about one in eight, or about 7.4 million women of reproductive age, have received help for infertility in their lifetime.[2] But when I tried to find information on men and infertility, it was much more difficult to find. I had to track it down. A study found that "approximately 50% of cases are due to women, and 20-30% of cases are due to men. The remaining 20- 30% of infertility cases is due to a combination of male and female factors,"[3] and the researchers discuss in detail how these cases are spread around the world, while explaining that it is very difficult to get accurate statistics overall. But the takeaway is that infertility can affect anyone.

So, what are the possible diagnoses? There are a lot. I will do a brief overview of many of them, but if you want to know more, I will cite where I got my information, as well as give suggestions at the end of this book for more reading material. Please note that this list cannot possibly outline every possible diagnosis, as there are so many. Every person's experience is very unique, so please, if the person you know and love has a very specific diagnoses, try to look into resources on your own if you are interested in learning more. The information below is partially from different articles[4] and partially from my personal experience and knowledge.

Male Factor Infertility

1. Azoospermia: In short, this means there is no sperm count. "It can be 'obstructive,' where there is a blockage preventing sperm from entering the ejaculate, or it can be 'nonobstructive' when it is due to decreased sperm production by the testis. Around 10 percent of infertile men and 1 percent of all men have azoospermia."[5]

2. Low motility: The motility is the movement of the sperm, and if that is low, the sperm may not be able to reach or penetrate the woman's egg.[6]

3. Low sperm count: If the sperm count is low, it decreases the odds that it will fertilize the woman's egg. An average number of sperm is about one hundred million per milliliter, and if the count is lower than fifteen to twenty million, a doctor will run more tests to confirm the low sperm count.[7]

4. Abnormal sperm: The sperm must be healthy and has to be carried into the semen to make it to the egg, and if there is an issue here, the sperm may be abnormal.[8]

Male factor infertility is even less discussed and understood than infertility overall, and there is a lot more to it than what have mentioned above. Overall, if there is male factor infertility there is a lot to consider when trying to get help and to see if it is possible for the person to have biological children. Many times, the couple or person will have to consider donor sperm which is a lot to consider on it's own. I wanted to explain some of the diagnoses around male infertility because people often assume it is the woman who has infertility issues, but it can be either or both partners, and it is difficult for people no matter who has the physical barriers to conceive. It is not anyone's business why a couple has issues, but it can helpful to know what they are going through.

Female Infertility

1. **Ovulation Diorders**
   - Polycystic ovary syndrome (PCOS): This causes a hormone imbalance, which affects ovulation. It is associated with insulin resistance and obesity, abnormal hair growth on the face or body, and acne, and it is the most common cause for female infertility.[9] There is also something called lean PCOS, which does not present itself in the same way as PCOS, but can equally impact a woman's fertility.
   - Premature ovarian failure: This is when an ovary no longer produces eggs, and it lowers estrogen production in women under the age of forty.
   - Hypothalamic dysfunction: Two hormones produced by the pituitary gland are responsible for stimulating ovulation each month—follicle-stimulating hormone (FSH) and luteinizing hormone (LH). Irregular or absent periods are the most common signs.[10]
2. **Problems with uterus or fallopian tubes**
   - Uterine fibroids: These are often benign but can interfere with implantation of the embryo.[11]
   - Damaged or blocked fallopian tubes: The eggs travel through the fallopian tubes and fertilize with the sperm to create an embryo, which becomes the baby. If the fallopian tubes are damaged or blocked, the egg cannot meet up with the sperm, making pregnancy impossible. It is usually caused by something that has happened, but for some people like myself, they are born with it.
   - Mayer-Rokitansky-Kuster-Hauser(MRKH) syndrome: This syndrome is when the uterus is underdeveloped or absent. It happens to about 1 in 4,500 women but is very unheard of.[12]
   - Cervical causes: Sometimes the cervix cannot produce the mucus to allow the sperm to travel to meet up with the egg. There can also be damage or cervical issues making it difficult for women to sustain pregnancies.[13]
   - Endometriosis: This is when tissue that normally

grows in the uterus grows and implants in other regions. This extra growth usually needs to be surgically removed, which can be risky. Endometriosis can also affect the lining of the uterus and make it difficult for an embryo to implant.[14] This is an extremely difficult disorder to identify—many women go years or decades without knowing what is causing their pain or infertility.

- Thin uterine lining: In order for a pregnancy to occur the embryo must implant into the uterine lining. Numerous studies have found that if a woman has a persistently thin uterine lining despite receiving adequate amounts of estrogen, then the chance for pregnancy is reduced. An optimal lining is seven to eight millimeters prior to an embryo transfer or embryo implantation.

- Asherman's syndrome: This is when there is scarring in the uterus, causing the front and back walls to stick together, making pregnancy very unlikely.[15]

3. **Past or current medications, treatments, and/or drugs**

- Chemotherapy and/or radiation: Cancer treatments, or treatments for similar medical conditions, can affect the fertility of women and men for the future. Doctors will usually discuss this with their patients prior to beginning treatments.

- Other: There are definitely more possible causes or diagnoses related to this category, and you can find more information about this in the resources listed later in this book.

4. **Genetic disorders**

Sometimes people have to do IVF, specifically with genetic testing, even if they can technically get pregnant naturally. They may not have any physical issues getting pregnant, but they may be carriers of genes that can cause miscarriages, loss in early childhood, or severe disabilities.

- Balanced translocation: A balanced or chromosomal translocation is a condition in which part of a chromosome has broken off and reattached in another location. In other words, it means that sections of two chromosomes have

switched places.
- Recessive genetic disorders: People can be carriers of genetic disorders that, while they do not present any symptoms themselves, have a chance of passing to a child. Many times, the pregnancy will appear fine, but the child may not live a very long life, sometimes less than a year.
- Chromosomal issues: Chromosomal issues can lead to early pregnancy loss, or very serious diseases.

5. **Secondary infertility**
   - Secondary infertility is the inability to become pregnant or carry a baby to term after previously giving birth to a baby. It shares many of the same causes of infertility. This can affect men and women.

6. **Unexplained infertility**
   - Sometimes a cause for infertility is never found. It can make it very difficult for people to know when to get treatment, or what kind of treatment to get.

* * *

Many infertility issues are considered "rare," but I believe this is skewed information. Once you know you have infertility issues, you are told again and again that you are an exception, that you are rare—but I do not believe these issues are actually as rare as people think. I think they just go undiagnosed, and there is not enough data or knowledge about infertility out there. For the actual possible diagnoses, the above information is just a very brief overview of many of the possible diagnoses, but this does not cover everything. For more information, see the recommended further resources at the end of the book.

What Are The Treatment Options?

Treatment options vary widely depending on the infertility diagnosis and what is available. It is also important to note that just because there is a certain treatment that could help, it does not mean that it is an option for someone, often for financial reasons. There are also personal or religious reasons that people do not seek out treatments. Other times, people make the decision to stop with treatments for their own mental health, as they cannot continue in the cycle of treatments anymore. And very importantly, just because someone does try a treatment option, it does not guarantee a child. There are unfortunately no guarantees, and people have to make the decisions to try options without knowing the outcome, just with the hope that it might give them the child they are yearning for.

As with the other sections of this chapter, this is just a brief overview of the treatment options, and I will include references and information of where to find more detailed information if you are interested.

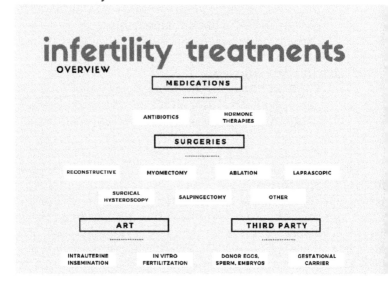

Medications

- Male factor infertility: antibiotics treat infections, erectile dysfunction, or premature ejaculation, hormone treatments help lower or raise hormones to improve function[16]
- PCOS: medications regulate cycle and help ovulate[17]
- Premature ovarian failure: hormone replacement therapy and other options help improve function, but overall this cannot be reversed[18]
- Hypothalamic dysfunction: hormone replacement therapy

- Fibroids: medications help break them up, but people often need more invasive options[19]
- Endometriosis: hormone therapy helps reduce or eliminate pain

Surgeries

- Male factor infertility: can correct or improve function
- Fibroids: myomectomy, laparoscopic surgery, ablation
- Damaged or blocked fallopian tubes: laparoscopic surgery, removal if the blocked tubes are affecting implantation
- Endometriosis: laparoscopic surgery can help remove endometriosis to improve chances of pregnancy, but this is often temporary; the most effective way to treat it is a hysterectomy, but this removes the uterus and ovaries and makes pregnancy and genetic children impossible, so many do not go this route unless absolutely necessary
- Asherman's syndrome: surgery is required to try to remove the adhesions, but success is not guaranteed.

Intrauterine Insemination

Intrauterine insemination (IUI) involves placing sperm inside a woman's uterus close to the fallopian tubes in order to increase the chances of conceiving.[20]
- Male factor infertility: "IUI is helpful in cases of male factor infertility because the sperm sample is specially prepared before it placed in the uterus."[21] This is a less invasive and less expensive option than IVF, but if a couple tries three cycles of IUI and does not get pregnant, it is usually recommended to move on to trying IVF.
  — Donor sperm: If a couple needs to use donor sperm, an IUI would be the least expensive and invasive option for pregnancy. The process is the same, except donor sperm is used instead of the partner's sperm.
- Cervical causes: The first choice of treatment for cervical factor infertility is an IUI because it avoids exposure of the sperm to the cervical mucus.[22]

In Vitro Fertilization

In vitro fertilization (IVF) is the most common assisted reproductive technology (ART) technique. IVF involves stimulating and retrieving multiple mature eggs, fertilizing them with sperm in a dish in a lab, and implanting the embryos in the uterus several days after fertilization. This is extremely simplified, but overall, if the process goes perfectly, it takes at least a few weeks to form the embryo(s). There is also an additional option of genetic testing and more, which is explained below.

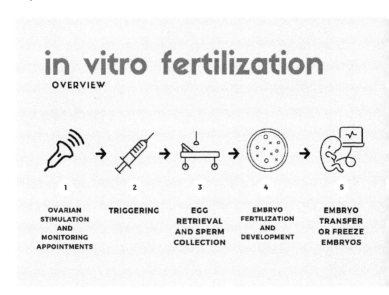

in vitro fertilization
OVERVIEW

1	2	3	4	5
OVARIAN STIMULATION AND MONITORING APPOINTMENTS	TRIGGERING	EGG RETRIEVAL AND SPERM COLLECTION	EMBRYO FERTILIZATION AND DEVELOPMENT	EMBRYO TRANSFER OR FREEZE EMBRYOS

IVF Optional Techniques

1. Surgical sperm aspiration: This is when sperm is surgically removed; usually only used when sperm count is very low.

2. Intracytoplasmic sperm injection (ICSI): A single healthy sperm is injected directly into a mature egg. ICSI is often used when there is poor semen quality or quantity, or if fertilization attempts during prior IVF cycles failed.[23]

3. Assisted hatching: This technique assists the implantation of the embryo into the lining of the uterus by opening the outer covering of the embryo (hatching).[24]

4. Genetic testing
   - Preimplantation genetic diagnosis (PGD): A technique that provides information about the gene makeup of the cells found in an embryo. An embryo biopsy removes about three to eight cells from each day five embryo (a blastocyst), and then cells are sent to a lab for testing. The embryo is usually frozen and implanted later. PGD can be used to identify approximately two thousand inherited single gene disorders and is 98 percent accurate at identifying affected and unaffected embryos.
   - Preimplantation genetic screening (PGS): Used to determine whether the cells in an embryo contain the normal number of chromosomes, which is forty-six. After an embryo grows in the lab, it is usually biopsied on day five (blastocyst stage). A few embryo cells are then sent to an external lab, which uses technology to count the number of chromosomes within each cell. Embryos with a normal number of chromosomes are "euploid," and those with an abnormal number are "aneuploid." The purpose of PGS is to avoid transferring an abnormal embryo into the uterus.[25]

5. Frozen embryo transfer (FET): When previously frozen embryos are thawed and transferred into the woman's uterus.[26] There are usually less medications involved than a fresh IVF transfer, and many doctors believe the success rates can be higher. This is based on a number of factors, but many people do opt for this.

6. Donor eggs or sperm
   - Most assisted reproductive technology is done using a couple's own eggs and sperm. However, if there are severe problems with either the eggs or the sperm, a couple or person may choose to use eggs, sperm, or embryos from a known or

anonymous donor.[27]

- For gay or lesbian couples, they must use donor eggs or sperm to have a child. For women, they have some options for pregnancy. If possible, they can do an IUI. If not, they can get IVF or reciprocal IVF. Reciprocal IVF is when one of the women has eggs retrieved, the eggs are combined with donor sperm, and the embryo is implanted into the other woman. For men, they must also use a surrogate or gestational carrier, along with donor eggs, for a child to be genetically related to one of the men

7. Embryo donation/adoption: This option utilizes embryos that were created by couples undergoing fertility treatment or from donor sperm and donor eggs specifically for the purpose of donation or adoption. This is an option if a couple wants to experience a pregnancy but cannot produce the embryos themselves. Just as with an adoption, once the couple adopts the embryos, they are legally their children.[28]

IVF by Diagnosis

- Male factor infertility: IVF with ICSI is usually the best option for male factor infertility. If the sperm count is very low or nonexistent, donor sperm will be recommended as well.
- Fallopian tube issues: For blocked or damaged fallopian tubes, IVF is often the best option. If a woman has no fallopian tubes - they can be damaged beyond repair or removed for another reason - IVF is the only option for pregnancy, as eggs cannot meet up with sperm naturally without a fallopian tube.[29]
- MRKH syndrome: Although there is currently no cure, IVF is an option if a woman has her ovaries, as eggs can still be retrieved. However, the couple will also need to use a gestational carrier, as this disorder causes the underdevelopment or absence of a uterus.
- Genetic issues: People who are carriers of specific genetic disorders often need to do IVF with genetic testing to ensure the best possible chance of a healthy

child.

IVF is necessary for many more people than listed here and s the most common form of assisted reproductive technology.

Gestational Carrier/Surrogate

A gestational carrier (GC), also called a gestational surrogate, occurs when a woman carries and delivers a child for another couple or person (intended parent[s]) according o a legally binding arrangement. Because the eggs will be retrieved from one woman and implanted in another, this echnique requires the use of IVF[30] or previously frozen embryos from past IVF cycle(s).

Here are a few more points about this type of fertility option:

- GCs are most often used by gay couples, as they cannot carry children themselves, but they are not the only ones who need GCs to have a child.
- Women with MRKH syndrome, as explained above, often need a GC to have a child, as they do not have a uterus.
- Women who have had a history of complications within their uterus or had to have a hysterectomy (the complete removal of the uterus) would have to use a GC.
- This is often recommended when a couple has tried many rounds of IVF with no success or recurrent pregnancy loss. Sometimes there is not a specific reason why a woman cannot get or stay pregnant, even if she has had a child in the past, and a GC is the best option for a healthy child.

Now, I am not putting adoption here as a "treatment" option because it is separate from infertility treatments, though it is a path that many people choose. Adoption is not an "easy fix" for infertility though; it is a personal decision, and it is also a long path. As I said earlier, this does not cover everything. For more information, see the recommended further reading at the end of the book.

What Can Be the Outcome of the Treatment Options?

Ideally, the outcome is obviously a healthy pregnancy and a healthy baby born from that pregnancy. Infertility treatments are about having a child, not just about getting pregnant. And ideally that is what happens! But unfortunately, many times that is not what happens, which is why infertility is so difficult People assume that treatments such as IVF are the final answer, a guarantee—and this is not true at all.

So what else can happen after a treatment?

For people taking medications, such as Clomid, the outcome can be a period and no pregnancy. This is devastating because they have been monitoring their cycle and inducing ovulation, and it feels that it just had to work. But it does not always. In fact, many times it does not work. Then they need to figure out what their next steps are, and where to go from there Medications for other fertility conditions, such as hormone replacement therapy, are also not guaranteed to work.

When surgery is used, the chance of success depends on the person, the diagnosis, and the severity of the diagnosis. For example, for endometriosis, after surgery has been done to remove all visible endometriosis, the likelihood of the disease recurring is estimated as 21.5 percent at two years and 40-50 percent at five years. Of this, around one third of cases will occur because some endometriosis has been missed at the original surgery.[31] This is just one example, but it shows that while surgeries can help achieve pregnancies and children they are not guaranteed or always permanent solutions to the infertility issues.

For people doing IUIs, success rates depend on the age and fertility health of both partners and can range anywhere from 2-20 percent each cycle, so it is important to know why the treatment is being considered and to take both partners into account to figure out a more accurate estimated success rate.[32] This is obviously a large range, but it just shows how much uncertainty and unknown there still is in infertility treatment.

and infertility overall. Nothing is guaranteed.

For people doing IVF, the overall success rates depend on a lot of factors as well, including the chosen clinic. A very general estimate states that about 27.3 percent of cycles are successful, and of those that are successful, about 81 percent result in a live birth.[33] These rates can be much higher or even lower depending on so many factors, so it is not really fair to focus on numbers. Overall, IVF is definitely not a guarantee.

In addition to the overall success rates, there are unfortunately negative outcomes that can happen along the way.

1. **Cancelled cycles**: A cycle can be cancelled, even once medication starts. While there is not a technical loss during a cancelled cycle, it is a loss of time and a loss of a potential pregnancy. Those suffering with infertility tend to think ahead about if it works, when they will get pregnant, and when a baby would be born, so it is devastating when a cycle is cancelled. This just means their future child is even farther away. There are multiple reasons a cycle can be cancelled—it can be because someone ovulates on their own too early or because their body is not responding to the medication correctly (for example, the uterine lining is not thick enough or there are not enough follicles to become potential eggs). And as of 2020, cycles have also been cancelled because of COVID-19 and offices shutting down temporarily. This is all out of our control, and it is incredibly painful. There is so much uncertainty and so much unknown, and this only extends timelines an unknown amount, which is very difficult to deal with.

2. **No viable eggs or embryos**: When someone is doing a full egg retrieval, there is the possibility that they will not get any eggs or embryos from the cycle. After all of the medications, time, surgery, and more, they could have nothing. Sometimes this means no viable eggs; other times it means no viable embryos. And even if the embryos are viable, they may not be genetically healthy. It is a numbers game—and for many, the numbers dwindle as time goes on, sometimes ending in zero embryos. This is extremely devastating because they

have to start completely from scratch. A full new round of IVF and another egg retrieval, all without knowing what the outcome will be. When this happens, people have to reevaluate and decide if they want to try again or find a new path.

3. **Ovarian hyperstimulation syndrome (OHSS)**: This is when the ovaries have been overstimulated and a transfer cannot immediately happen after the egg retrieval. This can be very painful and take a while to heal.

4. **Failed transfer**: This is when an embryo transfer does not work, but it is not the same as just getting a negative pregnancy test. It is an embryo that has been fought for, and a life that has been planned for. It is completely devastating and absolutely a loss. The best way I can explain is through this letter I wrote to the embryos we have lost (through failed transfers and miscarriages), which you can find on the next page.

5. **Ectopic pregnancy**: An ectopic pregnancy is when an embryo implants in the fallopian tubes instead of the uterus. This can happen naturally, through IUI, or through IVF. It is not a viable pregnancy and can be extremely dangerous. It often damages the fallopian tubes beyond repair, or the fallopian tube may have to be removed. This is also a loss because the baby is not viable, and the pregnancy has to end. And if a fallopian tube is affected or removed, there is even more to grieve, as this makes conception even more difficult for the future.

6. **Miscarriage**: Most people have heard of this, but this is when a pregnancy loss occurs. It most often happens in the first trimester but can happen later as well. The most common cause of miscarriages is when there is an abnormality in the embryo, but it can happen even with genetically tested embryos. Unfortunately, there is not just one type of miscarriage. Bleeding is often the first sign, but there is also something called a missed miscarriage, or blighted ovum, which is not diagnosed

until the first ultrasound when the baby has either stopped growing or has not grown at all. Miscarriages are incredibly painful, both physically and emotionally, in every single way. The number quoted for the rate of miscarriage is usually one in four, because on average across the whole population, and this is thought to be the overall rate. With that said, that is the estimated percentage of people who will experience only one miscarriage in their lives. Recurrent pregnancy loss, when more than one, and usually more than two, losses occur is much less common but is incredibly painful. It can feel like a healthy pregnancy will never be possible. And for people like me, sometimes this is the case.

It is important to note that options five and six listed above are not specific to IVF but can happen with IVF as well. These are just unfortunately negative possibilities when a woman does get pregnant. As with everything in this chapter, this is an overview of the potential options. It is definitely recommended to look into more details if you want to know even more about this.

Now, with all of this said, please do not talk to your friend and family member about all the negative possibilities from treatments. They are already terrified, and the last thing they need is for someone in their life to make them feel that their worries are justified. You should encourage them that it can work! I am explaining this to you more so that if someone does experience one or more of the negative outcomes above, you can better understand how devastating it is, and where they are coming from. And this can help you to support them better.

To help understand what it feels like to lose an embryo, even if there's technically no pregnancy, I have included a letter on the next page that I wrote after our fourth loss.

Dear embabies,

I grieve you. I miss you. I yearn for you.

I imagined a life for you, I've had dreams of your ultrasounds and holding you and feeding you — it felt so real I didn't want to wake up. Truthfully. I wanted to keep dreaming. It was perfect. But then I wake up. I wake up to a nightmare. A nightmare where you're not here. You're gone. Some gone before you're here — "failed transfer" — losses all the same. And some gone slightly later — miscarriage. Missed miscarriage. Chemical pregnancy. Nothing. Gone. Erased.

But not for me. You're forever etched, forever on my mind. I have pictures in my mind for how you would've looked, sounded, acted and I'm broken. I'm devastated. I'm at a loss — I'm lost. Why. Why me. Why always. Why never. I just can't understand — all I know is that I miss you before you even existed in real life — and so many cannot understand that loss. I'm a shell of who I once was.

Babies — you're all remembered for me.

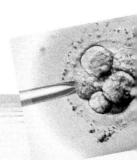

What Is the Financial Burden of Infertility?

This is subject to many factors, including where people live, their insurance policies, which policies the doctor's offices accept, and what types of treatments people are doing. There is a lot involved, but I will try to give a general look at the costs associated with infertility, as this is often something people forget. Unfortunately, in addition to the emotional and physical strain of infertility, the financial strain is huge too. It is often a barrier for people to have the child or children they want, simply because they cannot afford to do what they need to do to have children. I say this just so you can remember that sometimes people are not ending their treatments, or not pursuing treatments at all, by choice. Sometimes, they just literally cannot afford to continue.

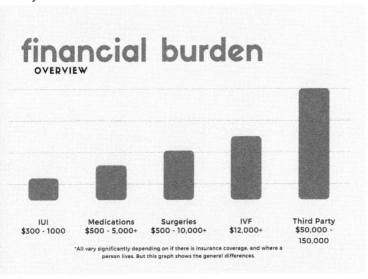

financial burden
OVERVIEW

IUI	Medications	Surgeries	IVF	Third Party
$300 - 1000	$500 - 5,000+	$500 - 10,000+	$12,000+	$50,000 - 150,000

*All vary significantly depending on if there is insurance coverage, and where a person lives. But this graph shows the general differences.

1. Medications: These costs can vary significantly. This is the most common type of treatment that insurance will cover, but insurance does not always cover medications. Depending on what is needed, the cost for medications can be covered completely or can cost in the thousands of dollars, and anywhere in between.

2. Surgeries: This is another one dependent on what insurance will cover. Similar to mediations, surgeries can be completely covered, there can be a limitation

on how many are covered, or they can be out of pocket, costing thousands of dollars.

3. IUI: Overall, each IUI cycle usually costs between three hundred to a thousand dollars out of pocket, and many people do not receive any fertility coverage.

4. IVF: The basic cost for IVF starts around twelve thousand dollars per cycle, but that does not include medication, which can be about five thousand dollars more. The additional tests also cost extra. ICSI costs about fourteen hundred to two thousand dollars, assisted hatching costs about four hundred to seven hundred dollars, and genetic testing can cost up to thirty-five hundred or more, with a limit on the number of embryos allowed to be tested, and extra cost for more. Freezing embryos costs up to one thousand dollars per year to keep stored, and every frozen embryo transfer cycle can cost about five thousand dollars or more. This does not include any additional surgeries or medications needed between these cycles. And remember, these are just for single cycles and many people do more than one, so the costs absolutely add up.

5. Gestational carrier: This varies greatly depending on where people live, who the GC is, and so forth. If the GC is a family member or friend, usually the medical costs are the main costs, which keeps the costs much lower. On the other end of the spectrum, it can cost couples up to one hundred and fifty thousand dollars or more to have a single child this way.[34]

Again, these are overviews and general information but they show that infertility has huge financial burdens for people, often inhibiting them from exploring the options they truly need.

What is an Infertility Resolution?

Many people assume that the only resolution to infertility is a child, but that is not always the case. There is more than one way for people to have infertility resolutions, and you should respect their decisions, no matter what they are.

infertility resolutions

Obviously after everything people go through to have children, the ideal resolution is a healthy pregnancy and child. People dealing with infertility will usually need medical help with this, as outlined above. For some, this means that the couple themselves is able to have the child, but for others, they need more help. If the woman is unable to carry a child herself, a couple may consider a gestational carrier or surrogate (GC). If one or both partners is not able to genetically have a child, the couple may consider donor eggs, donor sperm, or embryo adoption/donation. The couple can try to get pregnant themselves from here, or they may still need the help of a GC.

Other options that people may consider are adoption or fostering. These choices are very different from infertility treatments and have a long road of their own, but for many, this is the right way for them to try to complete their families. There are different guidelines for adoption depending on what state or country you live in and different ways to try to do it. For example, some couples will choose to go with an agency to help match them, and others will try to find someone themselves. Many agencies will require couples to stop any fertility treatments and focus solely on adoption, which can be a big choice on its own. There are also many things to consider when adopting, such as if you want an open adoption or closed adoption, which affects how much the birth parent would continue to be involved in the child's life. There are so many unknowns with adoption, and nothing is guaranteed. There is the extra pressure on people because it can take a very long time to be matched with a child, if ever, and the prospective parents have to decide on a variety of factors for a potential child, such as their age, background, gender, and more. People are often given very little notice if there is a child they can adopt, and even then, the process can feel nerve-wracking as they wait for things to finalize. There is much more about adoption than I can write here, so I have included a great website resource in the resources section of the book.[35]

Fostering a child is another path, and it is completely unique as well. There are qualifications that prospective parents need to meet, such as an age requirement, regular source of income, criminal background check, and more. There are also state requirements that vary, such as having a driver's license and configuring your house a certain way for safety purposes.[36] Additionally, the timelines are even more unknown. People can be told they are going to be taking a child in, only to have that change last minute. It also is not always certain how long a child will stay with a family, as the ultimate goal is usually to reunite them with their birth parents or family. There is sometimes an option for fostering to become an adoption, but this is not guaranteed and does not always happen. As with so much around infertility, there are huge psychological considerations for both fostering and adoption, and this is something people have to take into consideration when deciding to explore these paths.

The final option for some is to decide to live without children. This decision does not come lightly, but it can be the right decision for people. Again, this is their decision RESOLVE: The National Infertility Association words it very well: "Navigating the emotional journey towards being happy in a life without children involves a process of grieving. When individuals who have struggled with infertility face a life without children, it is usually by default. It is a loss of their dream. They often feel depressed, and their anguish is often rarely understood. Outsiders incorrectly assume that people living childfree have chosen not to have them."[37] RESOLVE goes on to explain that many people connect their value as a person to becoming a parent, which is only encouraged by society, so it can be hard for people to accept if they do not have children

No single resolution or answer is the right one, and every person's path is different and should be respected. Also, whether the person suffering has a child already or not does not make any of this any easier. Please do not remind them that they should be grateful if they already have children. They are grateful, trust me, more grateful than anyone could understand. But that does not take away from the pain, desire, and yearning for another child. And if they do not have any children, please stop asking when they will be having any—it s all they think about, and they have a right to privacy and to making their own decisions, when they can.

Additional Ways to Offer Support

Additional Ways to Offer Support

1   Help Advocate

One of the best resources to get involved with for infertility advocacy is RESOLVE: The National Infertility Association, but you can also advocate by making donations to different charities that offer infertility help. Or you can just advocate by simply helping to educate those around you.

2   Join A Walk

Just as with many other diseases, there are walks that happen throughout each year to raise money and awareness for infertility, as well as to advocate. This is a great way to get involved and support your loved one.

3   Send a Comforting Gift

Receiving something that is literally comfortable can be a wonderful surprise to someone experiencing infertility. Two of my personal favorite companies for this are:

- Uniquely Knitted: This organization serves people struggling with the emotional aspects of infertility in a variety of ways. The best way you can help is to donate to them directly, but if you want to send a comfortable gift to your friend or family member, they have boxes filled with so many wonderful things that will absolutely bring a smile to your loved one's face! The founders are infertility warriors themselves, so they know exactly what people need when they are struggling. Learn more at https://uniquelyknitted.org/.
- Cozy Warrior: This company makes some of the softest socks I have ever felt, and they are SO cozy! The

founders are also infertility warriors, and they aim to spread awareness and comfort with their socks. There is also a superstition that keeping your feet warm can help with fertility, so your loved one will appreciate this gift. Learn more at https://cozywarrior.org.

4   Do Some Further Reading

Although the prior chapter contains a lot of information, there is more to learn and understand. For a more in-depth look into researching infertility, here are some recommended readings. I have to note that these are not all of the available options for research, but simply what I have found helpful. I was not compensated for any recommendations in this book - just what I feel is most helpful.

Websites

RESOLVE: https://resolve.org
RESOLVE: The National Infertility Association allows you to learn more, take action, and shows people ideas for how to get help. I have personally organized a walk with them and cannot wait to be more involved with them in the future.

FertilityIQ: https://www.fertilityiq.com
This is a very informative website that has courses on infertility, as well as statistics and a lot more information about infertility overall.

Adoption.org: https://adoption.org
This website has so much information on adoption and fostering, from all different perspectives.

Creating A Family: https://creatingafamily.org
This company inspires adoptive, foster, and kinship parents and the professionals who support them.

Books

It Starts With the Egg *by Rebecca Fett*

This book is about how the science of egg quality can help you get pregnant naturally, prevent miscarriage, and improve your odds in IVF. This is extremely popular for people trying to conceive.

Had A Miscarriage *by Jessica Zucker*

Drawing from her psychological expertise and her work as the creator of the #IHadaMiscarriage campaign, this book is a heart-wrenching, thought-provoking, and validating book about navigating these spaces and the vitality of truth telling. She reminds us that it is very powerful to speak openly and unapologetically about the complexities of our lives.

Mackenzie's Mission *by Rachael Casella*

Like many other couples starting a family, Rachael and Jonathan had no idea they were both carriers for a genetic disease, and that one in twenty babies are affected by genetic birth defects. Their daughter was one of these babies, and Mackenzie's Mission is Rachael's beautiful and heartwarming account of Mackenzie's life, child loss, and a journey through IVF.

The Art of Waiting *by Belle Boggs*

Boggs takes her own struggle to conceive a child as a starting point for a wide-ranging, fascinating deep dive into the history, politics, and sociology of fertility. This is actually aimed toward people trying to understand infertility, rather than those experiencing it themselves.

Becoming *by Michelle Obama*

Something many people did not know about Obama before she wrote this book is how she and her husband struggled with miscarriages and infertility before having their children via IVF. She also talks about how infertility overall, and especially for black women and men, is often stigmatized and ignored.

We're Going to Need More Wine *by Gabrielle Union*

In this book, Union talks about her ongoing battle with recurrent pregnancy loss in addition to the ups and downs of being a black actor in white-centric Hollywood. She also talks about being a black woman with infertility, and eventually having a child through surrogacy.

5   Follow Social Media Accounts

See what people are saying, what they need, and what they ask for on social media—there's a lot of information there too. It is another form of research, and it is ongoing. Overall, the largest social media infertility communities are on Instagram. There are so many good accounts out there, but this is a starter list of who to follow.

@wheneverybodymatters

This is my page. I started it in 2019, while seeking out support and a new community, but it grew into more than I ever imagined. This page is part of what has encouraged and led me to write this book, and I will continue to keep updated information on it.

@the.ivf.warrior

Cheryl started one of the original and most followed infertility accounts. She helps spread awareness and community, and she is incredible! Follow along.

@missconceptioncoach

Chiemi is a counselor based in Canada and uses her knowledge and personal experience to help make people feel less alone when experiencing infertility. She spreads so much awareness and information daily.

@ihadamiscarriage

Jessica is a psychologist who specializes in reproductive and maternal health, and she created a campaign called #ihadamiscarriage to help raise awareness and end the stigma around having a miscarriage.

@pregnantish

Founded by Andrea, it is the first media site that helps people navigate the challenges of infertility and fertility treatments.

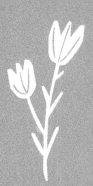

allow yourself
to learn about
others so your
empathy can
grow

Resources

Resources

1   https://www.who.int/reproductivehealth/publications/
infertility/art_ terminology2/en/
2   https://www.cdc.gov/nchs/fastats/infertility.htm
3   https://doi.org/10.1186/s12958-015-0032-1
4   https://www.medicalnewstoday.com/
articles/165748#outlook
5   https://www.hopkinsmedicine.org/health/conditions-
and-diseases/ azoospermia
6   https://www.hopkinsmedicine.org/health/conditions-
and-diseases/ azoospermia
7   https://www.hopkinsmedicine.org/health/conditions-
and-diseases/ azoospermia
8   https://www.mayoclinic.org/diseases-conditions/male-
infertility/ symptoms-causes/syc-20374773#:~:text=In%20
over%20a%20third%20 of,role%20in%20causing%20male%20
infertility
9   https://www.mayoclinic.org/diseases-
conditions/female- infertility/symptoms-causes/
syc-20354308#:~:text=Ovulation%20 disorders%2C%20
meaning%20you%20ovulate,Polycystic%20ovary%20
syndrome%20(PCOS)
10   https://www.mayoclinic.org/diseases-
conditions/female- infertility/symptoms-causes/
syc-20354308#:~:text=Ovulation%20 disorders%2C%20
meaning%20you%20ovulate,Polycystic%20ovary%20
syndrome%20(PCOS)
11   https://www.mayoclinic.org/diseases-
conditions/female- infertility/symptoms-causes/
syc-20354308#:~:text=Ovulation%20 disorders%2C%20
meaning%20you%20ovulate,Polycystic%20ovary%20
syndrome%20(PCOS)
12   https://ghr.nlm.nih.gov/condition/mayer-rokitansky-
kuster-hauser- syndrome#
13   https://www.mayoclinic.org/diseases-
conditions/female- infertility/symptoms-causes/
syc-20354308#:~:text=Ovulation%20 disorders%2C%20
meaning%20you%20ovulate,Polycystic%20ovary%20
syndrome%20(PCOS)

14   https://www.mayoclinic.org/diseases-conditions/female- infertility/symptoms-causes/syc-20354308#:~:text=Ovulation%20 disorders%2C%20 meaning%20you%20ovulate,Polycystic%20ovary%20 syndrome%20(PCOS)

15   https://my.clevelandclinic.org/health/ diseases/16561-ashermans- syndrome

16   https://www.mayoclinic.org/diseases-conditions/male-infertility/   diagnosis-treatment/drc-20374780

17   https://www.mayoclinic.org/diseases-conditions/pcos/diagnosis- treatment/drc-20353443

18   https://www.nichd.nih.gov/health/topics/poi/ conditioninfo/ treatments

19   https://www.mayoclinic.org/diseases-conditions/uterine-fibroids/ diagnosis-treatment/drc-20354294

20   https://www.lexico.com/en/definition/iui

21   https://www.shadygrovefertility.com/blog/ diagnosing-infertility/   overcoming-male-factor-infertility/

22   https://edmonton.pacificfertility.ca/our-resources/cervical- factor-infertility/#:~:text=The%20 first%20choice%20of%20   treatment,exposure%20 to%20the%20cervical%20mucus

23   https://www.mayoclinic.org/diseases-conditions/infertility/diagnosis-   treatment/drc-20354322

24   https://www.mayoclinic.org/diseases-conditions/infertility/diagnosis-   treatment/drc-20354322

25   https://www.arcfertility.com/ivf-pgd-pgs-genetic-testing-can-tell- embryo/

26   https://www.shadygrovefertility.com/blog/ treatments-and-success/ frequently-asked-questions-about-frozen-embryo-

27   https://www.mayoclinic.org/diseases-conditions/infertility/diagnosis-   treatment/drc-20354322

28   https://www.asrm.org/topics/topics-index/ embryo- donation/#:~:text=Embryo%20donation%20

is%20a%20procedure,a%20   researcher%20to%20further%20the

29   https://www.healthline.com/health/womens-health/blocked- fallopian-tubes#:~:text=If%20your%20 fallopian%20tubes%20   are,blockages%20may%20 not%20be%20possible

30   https://www.reproductivefacts.org/news-and-publications/patient-fact-sheets-and-booklets/documents/fact-sheets-and-info-booklets/   gestational-carrier-surrogate/#:~:text=A%20gestational%20carrier%20 (GC)%2C,not%20come%20from%20the%20carrier

31   https://medicalxpress.com/news/2018-09-surgery-endometriosis.   html#:~:text=Success%20 rates,missed%20at%20the%20original%20 surgery

32   https://www.shadygrovefertility.com/ treatments-success/basic-   treatments/intrauterine-insemination-iui

33   https://www.webmd.com/infertility-and-reproduction/guide/in- vitro-fertilization#2

34   https://surrogate.com/intended-parents/ the-surrogacy-process/   how-much-does-surrogacy-cost/#:~:text=According%20to%20their%20 website%2C%20the,program%20estimates%20 for%20unforeseen%20 developments

35   https://adoption.org/

36   http://www.families4children.com/fc_req.cfm

37   https://resolve.org/what-are-my-options/living-childfree/

About the Author

About the Author

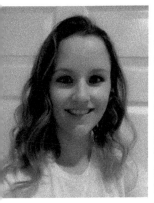

Alexandra is a first time author, who is passionate about spreading community, awareness, support. and advocacy for infertility. In 2015, she and her husband started trying to have children, and quickly realized they would need help, and that IVF would be their only option for children. They felt lucky when their first round of IVF gave them in their first son in 2017. Quickly after, Alexandra and her husband decided to try for another child, recognizing it could take some more time given her diagnoses. They had no idea what they were in store for.

Since 2017, they have had two cancelled cycles, two failed transfers, and two miscarriages. Alexandra has been diagnosed with many infertility issues, and eventually found out that she could no longer carry a pregnancy full term, even when IVF did work. Their final option for a second biological child was surrogacy. They matched with an incredible person, and finally had their second son at the end of 2020!

In 2019, Alexandra started an infertility Instagram blog to connect with others, but she had no idea what it would turn into. Not only does it allow her to connect with others, but also to advocate for herself and others, and get involved with the community as a whole. She has found that there is a lack of resources for those wanting to offer support and wrote this book in an effort to help make it easier for people to do so, without feeling so in the dark about how.

Alexandra would say that she is a part of a club no one wants to belong to, but the members are absolutely incredible. And she is immensely proud and honored to be able to have her Instagram blog, website, and this book, to help in any way she can!